Exercises for Thinking Mindfully: Volume Six

Mindfulness Practices for Persons with Parkinson's Disease

9/3/2014
Parkinsons Recovery
Robert Rodgers PhD

Contents

The Parkinsons Recovery Mindfulness Series

Realistically speaking, how can the intense level of stress that aggravates the symptoms of Parkinson's disease be calmed? Better yet, how can they be quieted? My research over the past decade reveals that using your mind to drop the stress level down a notch or two always backfires. When you tell yourself:

- *Settle down!*
- *Take it easy!*
- *Stop being so stressed out!*

The stress level ratchets up, not down. Attempts to force the stress and anxiety levels to adjust downward induce an internally generated stress. They pile more stress on top of an excess of stress that already exists. There are certainly a sufficient number of external generators of stress in every one's life. Why infuse more stress that you create yourself, even with the best of intentions?

If the mind is not a useful technique to reduce stress, what is? The most eloquent answer I have for you is to become more mindful of what is experienced in the present moment. Becoming more mindful shifts you into the experience of the "now" which in itself is less stressful (unless you have been kidnapped by terrorists!).

It is stressful to anticipate events you imagine will occur in the future. The events we imagine rarely happen. Does this ring true for you? We all create unnecessary stress in our lives by how and where we focus our thoughts and attention.

It is stressful to agonize over the past. When we think about the past, we are much more likely to think about unpleasant experiences that induce stress. The past event itself was traumatic enough. Yet, we insist on reliving the trauma over and over again through our memories. It seems some of us just can't get enough stress in our lives.

The problem with upping the ante on stress levels is that – as you well know – symptoms of Parkinson's disease become worse. When you are not as stressed, your symptoms are far less problematic.

I have reached one solid conclusion from my ten years of research on Parkinson's disease. Symptoms will drive you crazy when you are stressed and are far less problematic when stress is under control.

Now, if you can't use your mind to become more mindful (which creates added stress in itself) how in the world can you quiet down a frantic lifestyle? I have concluded that the simplest and most effective solution to reducing stress levels is to become more mindful.

The transformation is possible step by step through these simple exercises you can do anywhere, anytime of the day. The Parkinsons Recovery mindfulness exercises are designed to focus your attention on the present moment as attention on either the past or the future is diverted. A renewed focus on the present moment reduces stress levels. Mindfulness is a lifestyle that will reduce stresses in your life if you set the intention to take a mindfulness practice seriously.

I recommend that you practice each of the exercises for a week or longer. Incorporate each practice into your regular routines and habits. Attempts to do all of the exercises simultaneously will likely induce more stress which – obviously – is contrary to the intent of a successful mindfulness program.

Give each exercise a little time and space. Invite the stresses in your life to dissipate. Allow the experience of each practice to engulf you. In so doing, watch the stresses in your life dip down to new lows along with a concurrent relief of any and all symptoms that you have currently been experiencing.

This volume is one out of nine I have developed to support the recovery of persons who currently experience neurological symptoms. A full listing of the Parkinsons Recovery Mindfulness themes follows:

Exercises for Thinking Mindfully
Mindfulness Practices for Persons with Parkinson's Disease
Volume Six

Robert Rodgers, PhD

Parkinsons Recovery

www.parkinsonsrecovery.me

Olympia, Washington

Thoughts

Since you saw the title of this mindfulness challenge this week, how many thoughts have rattled through your mind: five, ten, even fifteen? We process at least 60,000 thoughts that rattle throughout our minds each and every day.

As it turns out, the big surprise is that 90% of those thoughts are the same thoughts. If we dump out thoughts that are not in our best and highest good - thoughts that are negative and thus have very low energetic charges - we free up a massive storage capacity in our energetic hard drive. With a renewed processing capacity, we are magically able to do what it is that we want to do with our lives and manifest our destiny so-to-speak. How then can we track the 60,000 thoughts that rattle through the hamster wheel in our minds each and every day?

The mindfulness challenge this week requires use of a little technology and a little preparation. My invitation is to set a timer at a set time sequence each and every day. Find a timer that might be on your cell phone or smart phone or watch. Perhaps you might want to use a timer in your kitchen that can be set for a fixed number of minutes. Set the timer that you select to use for 54 minutes.

Each and every time the timer buzzes (whether the timer is your smart phone, cell phone, watch or timer from the kitchen) stop and note whether or not the thought that you are having when the buzzer rang is a positive thought, a neutral thought or a negative thought. Positive thoughts give you energy. Neutral thoughts have a flat energetic charge. Negative thoughts deflate your energy.

The other technology you will need for the week is a small notebook and pen or pencil that you can carry around with you in your pocket or somewhere close at hand. Every time the buzzer goes off – every 54 minutes – all you have to do is stop what you are doing. Acknowledge what it was that you happened to be thinking at that particular moment. Do not bother recording the specifics of the thought. That will take too much time and is totally unnecessary.

All you want to do every 54 minutes is to acknowledge the thought you were having when the buzzer went off and then place a single mark on your notebook; a plus sign for a positive thought, a dash for a neutral thought and a minus sign for a negative thought. By the end of the day (if you have succeeded in recording a thought every 54 minutes) you are going to have anywhere from 8 to 12 counts showing how many thoughts (at the 54 minute mark) were positive, neutral and negative. And of course, you will have a report for each day of the week!

Set your timer today for 54 minutes. Feel free to alter the time lapse between when the buzzer goes off from one day to the next. Tomorrow set the timer to an hour and ten minutes or set it to 34 minutes. Set the timer to whatever time sequence seems appropriate. It depends in part on how often you are willing to be interrupted during the day. Or of course, you can just keep it set at 54 minutes each day this week.

Just remember to code each thought as positive, neutral or negative each and every time the buzzer goes off. One note of caution: Be sure to turn the timer off when you go to sleep because you don't want to be waking up and coding your dreams.

This will take a bit of effort to prepare. It does take a little time in terms of actually recording the energy of your thoughts throughout the day. I promise, however, that it will give you incredible insights on the proportion of thoughts that are enriching your life force and those that are not.

Have a fun time this week as you monitor the quality of your thoughts.

Deeper Meaning Behind Thoughts

At the core of the recovery process lays the pattern of our thoughts. If our thoughts are dominated by negativity, it is unlikely that we have much promise of recovering.

I now invite you to analyze the reports of your thoughts that you recorded in your notebook over the past few days.

1. First, tally up the total number thoughts that you recorded (whether they were positive, neutral or negative).
2. Second, count the number of instances you recorded a positive thought.
3. Third, calculate the proportion of positive thoughts by dividing the number of positive thoughts by the number of total thoughts. This will yield a proportion.
4. Fourth - multiply this proportion by 100 so you have a percent that ranges between 0% and 100%.

It is possible that if you are in a particularly bad mood, this proportion could conceivably be 0%. It happens to everyone.

What is the result? Is the proportion of thoughts that are positive that you just calculated only 10%? If so, the probability, the possibility, the inevitability of your

9

recovery turns out to be very, very small. I say this even if you are taking positive action on many fronts with regard to therapies and other modalities that research shows help reverse symptoms.

Our thoughts lay at the foundation of everything that happens in our lives. If we are inundated with negative thoughts, our cells, muscles, tissues and neurons will be assaulted as if we were in a war zone. Negative thoughts do us no good whatsoever. Worse, they ultimately kill cells that are healthy. Positive thoughts, on the other hand, have an incredibly high energetic charge; they are the source of all healing. They sustain and create healthy cells.

To acknowledge the proportion of positive thoughts offers a good indication of work that you might consider doing to transform negativity. Everyone has negative thoughts. The challenge to health turns on situations where the negative thoughts dominate your thought patterns.

Becoming an individual who has mostly positive thoughts means that the actions and steps that you take to help recover from the neurological challenges that you currently experience will in fact take full effect.

For example, perhaps you have decided to pursue a strategy of eating an organic diet of vegetables and fruits. If you are also having positive thoughts in the vicinity of 90% or 95%, this strategy should yield the maximum effect possible. If you are eating healthy, raw foods and your thoughts are more in the realm of 10% positive, the end result of eating healthy foods will not have a full effect. It will be significantly diminished.

Bolster efforts that you are currently pursuing to help your body heal by closely monitoring the energetic charge of your thoughts. Acknowledge the extent to which the proportion of positive thoughts may not be as high as you would wish (if that is the case). Take positive action to banish all of those negative, repetitive thoughts that are not in your best and highest interest.

Negative thoughts rattle around the hamster wheel of our minds over and over each day. By the end of the day, we have actually had the same negative and damaging thought as many as 5,000 or 10,000 times in a single day alone. I know this to be true because I have tracked my own thoughts!

1. Eliminate the damaging effect of negative thoughts.
2. Replace them with positive ones.

Flood yourself with the energy necessary to manifest your heart's desire. Become mindful throughout the day of each and every thought that enters into your mind; especially those that you're having when that buzzer rings off. Set the intention to transform negativity into thoughts that are in your best and highest good. Celebrate a recovery that begins to accelerate.

Be Kind to Your Body

The mindfulness challenge this week shifts from the silly and the funny and the specific to a more somber and quite profound assignment. The invitation is to be kind to your body. Before I explain how I suggest that you accomplish this task, let me explain the idea behind being kind to your body.

When symptoms flare we can very easily get very angry and upset at our body, even to the point of wanting to occupy another body. These low-vibration thoughts are certainly not in our best and highest good and certainly not in our body's best and highest good. Let me explain the dynamic that is involved. First, I need to spin a story.

> When I was ten years old my father, mother and my two brothers took a brief two-week vacation to Daytona Beach, Florida. I have quite vivid memories of this trip because while driving down to Florida from Atlanta my father was in a particularly ornery and mean mood. Talking to my mother (oblivious to the fact that we were all in back seat of the car) he ranted and raved about how he wished he had never had children. They were too much trouble. They were a huge expense. They were a pain in the ass. This went on and on throughout our entire trip from Atlanta, Georgia to

12

Daytona, Florida. Of course my brothers and I felt absolutely awful.

Using this experience as a template we will simply make a short transformation. Think about the possibility that instead of my whole self being present in the car, only my body occupies the back seat of the car. The words from my father in the front seat are actually words I am saying to my body which occupies the back seat of the car. In effect, I am saying cruel things to my own body.

Can you imagine how my body actually feels? It too will feel absolutely horrible. That certainly is not conducive to health, wellness and balance.

One more example – it is important that you get the gist of what I am talking about. Imagine that your body is your loved pet - whether a dog, a cat, a horse, a parakeet or a hamster – a loved pet that was near and dear to you as a child, as a teenager, as a young adult or is near and dear to you now. Imagine how that pet would feel if you sling negative thoughts at them. Let me reiterate so you just get an idea of how horrible all of this really can be. Just imagine you have your loved pet on a leash and you have the following conversation with them:

> *"You're just not working very well these days. I do not like cleaning up your messes. I'm really very disappointed in you. It seems day in and day out you have these awful problems. I'm tired of dealing*

13

with this problem and quite frankly, I'd like to have another pet. I'm just sick of it. I want this to be over with. I want you to get well and I want you to do it quickly. I'm sick and tired of having look at you."

Now, put yourself in the position of the pet. The pet obviously is going to feel pretty horrible. Most pets really do understand what we say. But, even if they do not understand the cognitive meaning of these words they will most certainly feel the energetic assault of negativity.

We may be able to get another pet but the body we occupy is all we get. There is no body exchange store. We can't exchange our body for another one. If we insist on treating it with just these types of accusations and this horrible negativity, our body is not going to respond well no matter what steps we take to help it heal. .

The challenge this week is to shift our orientation. Of course, our negative thoughts come from an unconscious place from long ago and far away. Of course, they tend to be habitual and repetitive. Most people with Parkinson's have an unconscious habit of abusing their body with negative thoughts because it is working "normally."

This week shift any and all negative energy to a positive energy of kindness toward your body. In the morning when you get up and in the evening before you go to bed, I have an invitation to you. Say to your body,

May you be free from discomfort.

May you be at ease.

May you come into a full balance.

May you be healthy.

May you be centered.

May you be balanced.

May you be calm and at ease.

Thank you for always being there for me.

Thank you for all that you do for me.

Of course what you say to your body will come from your heart and will not necessarily reflect the words above. It is quite sufficient when you see yourself in the mirror in the morning and when you see yourself in the mirror in the evening, to simply look at yourself with an open heart say,

"Thank you for all that you do for me."

Be kind to your body this week when you get up in the morning and when you go to bed at night. At other times during the day—send that loving energy to the one that needs it the most right now - your precious body that is doing its best to heal.

Deeper Meaning Behind Being Kind to Your Body

Many people find it particularly difficult to actually remember to be kind to their bodies twice a day—once in the morning and once before they go to bed. Has this been the case for you?

Since receiving this invitation, how many times each day have you been kind to your body – zero, one, two, five, ten, twenty? How many times? Why is it so easy to forget to be kind to our body? There are many reasons of course but some of those reasons fall under the rubric of images that we see of body types that are supposed to be ideal; movie actors, athletes, models, you name it.

If you will just step back however, ask yourself the question,

> *"What have these famous persons done to their bodies in order for them to take the particular shape that we see?"*

Many models starve themselves with anorexia and risk death. Many athletes take steroids. They tend to have early deaths because they have abused their bodies so horribly. Many actors have painful facelifts that impose significant trauma to a body. These are the ideal body types I ask you? I don't think so.

What criticisms do you have of your own body? Face up to it. Of course, you are only talking to yourself. You are only making a confession that you can hear now. What criticisms do you have?

Are your legs too short?
Is your belly too fat?
Are your breasts too small or large?
Is your hair too wiry or too gray?
Do you have too many wrinkles?
Do you have flab under chin?
Are you muscles like spaghetti?

What are your criticisms? Have I landed on any that resonate with you? You see, all of these are only judgments of our body – our one and only body - that actually performs miracles for us day in and day out.

The key idea here is that our bodies cannot thrive or heal if stuck in a war zone bunker where the bullets are negative thoughts. Nothing can thrive under unrelenting criticisms that damage the cells and tissues of our precious bodies. Children cannot survive these types of insults and attacks. Pets certainly cannot survive them.

And by the way, potted plants cannot either! When we present workshops, we will often bring two potted plants. One of them, we invite people to be kind to. The other we invite people to ignore. At the end of just two days, guess which plant is withering away?

17

As it turns out the mindfulness task of being kind to your body is worth far more than any medicine, surgery or therapy of any origin or cost. Some people believe being kind to your body is a selfish act. Let me clue you in. If you cannot honestly and genuinely be thoroughly loving and kind to your own body, it will not be possible for you to offer genuine kindness to others. If you wish is to be of service to others, the best way to learn how to offer meaningful service is to be kind to this precious vehicle that you occupy—this vehicle of your body - day in and day out - even when it does not seem to be functioning quite the way you would prefer.

- *Honor your body.*
- *Treasure your body.*
- *Thank your body day in and day out for all that it does for you.*

Be patient. Your body will, in due time, show its appreciation for all of your kindnesses.

Gratitude

The invitation this week is to fill your heart, soul and body with gratitude each and every day. Here is how to go about doing just that.

Place beside your bed a sheet of paper or even a journal as well as a pen or pencil. This exercise will take only five minutes every day.

Before you go to sleep, retrieve the piece of paper beside your bed (or your journal) and the writing instrument. Reflect back on the day you have just finished living. Write a notation of three experiences that you are grateful for having that day. Do this every day.

Experiences you record do not have to be big deals. They might consist of a passing moment in time; a smell that you appreciated, a look from a stranger; a comment from a friend or a loved one; a compliment; a special way that you happened to feel earlier in the day even if only for a few minutes.

Do not make this exercise a big deal. You will not do it if you do make it a big deal. Make it a small task. At the end of the day, take out the paper and pen or pencil and enter a short and sweet notation that answers the question, "What have I been grateful for today?"

19

There is no screening or decision making involved here. There is certainly no editing required. Simply make a note of whatever comes first to your mind.

1. *Experience one*
2. *Experience two*
3. *Experience three*

Record whatever you are grateful for - big events or tiny events. Whatever first comes to mind. You can always add to the list if you wish.

- *It may be certain memories you are grateful for.*
- *It may be certain thoughts.*
- *It may be a certain feeling.*
- *It may be a message your body is communicating to you that has been a welcome, delightful gift.*

Whatever you are grateful for note it on your paper at the end of the day. Do it every day. We are talking here about taking five minutes each day. Becoming mindfully grateful can fill your days with an abundance of joy and happiness.

Enjoy being grateful this week. Be grateful you are being grateful!

Deeper Meaning Behind Being Grateful

We all have a choice moment to moment with regard to how we live our life. We may choose to immerse ourselves into the negative aspects of all that is going on. The news media is particularly adept at spinning negative stories. Pick up any newspaper or listen to any television station or report of the news on any day. It will be filled with negative, depressing stories.

It is also very easy to get mired into a very negative state of mind with regard to what your body might be communicating to you. Perhaps we are thinking today that:

> *"My symptoms are flaring up today. I will likely feel worse tomorrow."*

When we churn the same negative thoughts around and around a hamster wheel of our own creation, we feed into the energy of negativity which is bound to fuel the symptoms. The key to healing from the inside-out is to transform the repetitive negative thoughts that haunt us day in and day out. The key to recovery is to maintain a positive frame of mind each and every moment of our lives.

21

My questions are these. You have been keeping a written record of what you have been grateful for each and every day? As the days have progressed, have you wanted to add more than just three items to your list? Perhaps you did. On the second or third day perhaps you added a fourth and a fifth reason to be grateful to the basic list of three.

Have you noticed that when you experienced something pleasurable during the day you thought to yourself:

> *"Ah, that's something I want to add to my list*
> *tonight before I go to bed?"*

See what kicks in when we begin to make a habit of maintaining a positive attitude, a positive state of mind? It escalates into having more and more positive thoughts and more and more positive experiences. It reduces depression significantly. Best of all, it fuels the pleasure of happiness throughout the day.

When we honor and relish the positive experiences of our life, we feed into the positive energy that makes the manifestation of recovery possible. When we nurture positive thoughts of gratitude we create an energy that is conducive to healing and wellness. We may say to ourselves,

"But wait a minute, I've got to be sure that I am prepared for the future."

When you have those thoughts, what are you really saying to yourself? You're likely saying,

"Oh, yeah, that is right, I'm going to be disabled in a few years so I need to do some planning."

That thought is destined to steer you straight into a nursing home. Is that what you really want? Or, do you want to live a vibrant, free, active life that has a force and an energy that is limitless? Be mindfully grateful for each and every moment of your life.

We tend to remember and relish only negative experiences, not positive ones. We go back into the past and say to ourselves,

"I wish I had done this and that. Matters wouldn't have turned sour if I had acted differently."

Those thoughts are not going to change anything. The past is past.

The way to change our health and wellness is to live moment to moment, to be mindful and live in the present. The origins of negative thoughts reside in past memories or future fantasies. It is tough to create negative thoughts when we are mindful of enjoying the present moment.

23

You are cordially invited to continue keeping your list of what you are grateful for at the end of each day. Continue to acknowledge that there are many glorious, positive experiences that you are having each and every day.

Allow your list to expand beyond the count of three if you so wish. Constrict yourself not. Allow yourself to add more and more experiences, thoughts and actions that you are grateful for each and every day as the week progresses.

I suggest to you, whether you decide to continue the list or not, it is very likely you will be thinking to yourself,

> *"Ah, that's something that I could add to my list before I go to bed tonight."*

Once you have turned on the flow of positive thoughts it is virtually impossible to shut them down. Isn't that cool?

Feel the positive life force surge within your body. Observe your symptoms dissolve.

May you have a magnificent week as you find yourself being grateful for the magnificence of living life to the fullest.

News Fast

After many years of focusing my attention exclusively on the factors that contribute to the symptoms of Parkinson's disease, I have two truths to offer.

The first truth is – **Change is necessary to heal.** There is an imbalance in your body that is creating the neurological symptoms associated with the diagnosis of Parkinson's disease. If you are serious about reversing those symptoms, you will have to make some changes in your behavior. I fully recognize this is a broad statement which implies a variety of possibilities:

- *Change may mean changes in how you are making decisions about what to do each day.*
- *Change may mean making changes about how you live your life.*
- *Change may mean how you move your body.*
- *Change may mean what you put in your body.*

Whatever the nature of the change that is required, something has to shift if you expect that neurological symptoms will resolve and reverse.

The second truth is - **Stress has a direct connection to the symptoms.** When people are stressed the symptoms

25

flare. When people are joyously pursuing their life's passion, symptoms are hardly even noticeable.

Have you ever heard the statement:

"Fasting is good for you?"

The challenge this week may be difficult for some of you, but I am going to suggest a fast. Not a food fast (although research does show that a food fast reduces symptoms), not a people fast, but a news media fast.

Are you a news junkie? If so, this particular challenge may be particularly onerous and difficult. Permit me to suggest it anyway. Your life may be transformed if you accept this challenge.

What does this fast entail for you to become more mindful moment to moment during the week?

1. **No watching TV of any type.**
2. **No reading newspapers from any source.**
3. **No listening to the radio.**

If you count up the hours that you spend devoting attention to those three media sources, you may be surprised at how much of your life you are spending being exposed to the propaganda of the mass media. I have personally realized that much of which is advertised to be news is actually just propaganda of one type or another. So, why even bother?

Once you turn off the TV, once you stop reading the newspaper, once you turn off your radio (or never turn the radio on) what are the alternatives? What do you do instead? There are many options. Let me suggest a few.

- *Play a musical instrument*
- *Learn how to play a musical instrument you have always wanted to learn.*
- *Listen to music.*
- *Cook.*
- *Chill out and relax.*
- *Meditate.*
- *Walk.*
- *Exercise.*
- *Paint.*
- *Write.*
- *Dream.*
- *Talk with friends and family over the phone.*
- *Invite neighbors over to sit on your porch or your back deck and hang out.*

Of course the list of alternatives is endless. Gardening may be one of your favorites. Whatever the choice might be, the key is, turn off mass media for this week. Monitor how you are feeling and be aware of your stress level. May you have fun with the challenge of this news media fast this week.

27

Deeper Meaning Behind a News Fast

What is the deeper meaning behind cutting yourself off from all mass media? Let me first speak to that question by talking briefly about my own personal experience.

When in my twenties I served as a navy officer in the Roosevelt Roads Navy Station in Puerto Rico. There was no television to be seen in Puerto Rico at that time. I really had no choice but to experience a news fast of all types for three years while serving in the US Navy.

When returning to the United States, I naturally turned on the TV to see what I had missed while I was away. After watching a few days my reaction was that I had not missed anything of any great importance. I continued nonetheless to watch the news over the next 20 or so years at which point I decided to conduct a media fast for myself. I have not now actually watched TV for several decades other than when I happen to be staying in a hotel room and want to chill out.

The level of my anxiety and stress has been profoundly reduced as a result of not being exposed to the mass media in the form of television, in the form of newspapers and in the form of radio. Because my stress level has been significantly reduced moment to moment, my health has been excellent.

Why has my own news fast had such a positive impact on my health and my well-being? I think it is because the mass media conveys information that instantly creates anxiety and stress. Both are directly connected to the symptoms of Parkinson's. It makes good sense to me to do anything possible to reduce any and all stimuli that enhance and provoke stress and anxiety. When watching the news media or listening to the radio or reading the newspaper, we are exposing ourselves to horrendous information and images. Stories of gloom and doom dominate the mass media.

What do we see on the TV when we watch? We see information about crimes, about assaults, about terrorism, about death, about court proceedings, about animal cruelty, about negative political advertising, about sheer propaganda, lies, suffering, pain, lawsuits, gangs, scare tactics, the world is coming to an end; the list really is endless. Think back on any TV program that you might have recently watched. What positive and uplifting story did you watch?

When I am at a hotel staying overnight and surf television stations I quite frankly become depressed. I ask myself why am I wasting my time surfing these TV channels when there are no uplifting programs to watch?

As I suggested at the outset, change must be taken if you expect to see the reversal of symptoms. What change is required? Consider a news fast to be one important

29

possibility. The end goal is to reduce stress and anxiety in your life. One simple way to accomplish this goal is to go on a news fast, not just this week, but how about for the rest of your life?

If you pursue this particular mindfulness challenge, I suggest that you monitor your symptoms along with your levels of stress and anxiety. If your experience is like mine you will indeed discover that you are significantly less stressed. When you are less anxious, you afford an opportunity for the imbalances that may be present in your body to resolve naturally, with no side-effects, comfortably, effortlessly.

Making this change in your life style requires no prescription medications, no visits to doctors and no listening to Parkinsons Recovery radio shows. It simply means that you change your behavior. Instead of exposing yourself to the horrors of the world, take alternative action that is in your best and highest good. Pursue passions that are deeply fulfilling rather than profoundly depressing.

Many people are resistant to undertake and accept the challenge of a news fast. They feel as though they will miss something important. I am here to tell you that there is no way this can happen if you go on a news fast (having been on one now for over a decade). When something significant happens in the world, you will hear about it very, very quickly. It is really quite amazing. People will be talking about it. It is very evident from any encounter with anyone anywhere, whether they be strangers or friends. The news will be in your face. People will say:

"Have you heard?"

And the simple answer is:

"No. Tell me about it."

You will get the full report – usually in great detail - of the event which just occurred.

Rest assured, you are not going to miss anything. You will hear about it anyway. Better yet, if there is a horrendous event in the world, you will not expose yourself to the horrors of the images. After all, if there is a horrendous event in the world, what can you personally do about it?

If this is part of your job, of course you must see and know and do and go to the place where the horrendous event occurred. For most of us, we can do nothing to help out those who are suffering from the earthquakes or the tsunamis or the hurricanes or the tornadoes. We are too far distant and unable to provide any assistance.

What do we get if we actually expose ourselves to the information and the images and the sounds that are connected to disasters? What we get is an assault into the tissues of our body of trauma. This creates stress and

31

anxiety. What do you get in return? Symptoms become much, much worse.

So, what do you really get out of spending time watching TV? You spend time watching the horrors of the world.

1. *Do you get better?*
2. *Do you feel better?*

The answer is no; just the reverse. You will feel worse, less able to help out others when they are in need when you happen to be in a position to help.

In summary, I say to you the following. I have personally found that a news fast has provided extreme benefits to me over the last several decades. Try it out at least for a week. See what happens with you. It is amazing to me to watch how much negativity is conveyed in the mass media. It is also exciting to discover how much time is freed up when you stop spending your time allowing the mass media to gobble up your energy.

Have fun with your news fast. I hope you continue to accept the challenge—no TV, no reading newspapers, no listening to the radio. Engage alternative actions. Make a change in your life. Celebrate what happens with your symptoms.

Has your work on these exercises been stress free? Has it been helpful in reducing your symptoms? I certainly hope so! This is the primary reason I developed the mindfulness exercises in the first place.

If you struggled with pacing out these mindfulness exercises so as not to induce more stress, there are several Parkinsons Recovery programs that might help expedite your recovery. My Parkinsons Recovery Mindfulness Program sends the mindfulness exercises in an email to you each and every week. The initial exercise is sent to your email address on day one of the week and the deeper implications are sent four days later. The Parkinsons Recovery Mindfulness Program takes one full year to complete as each exercise is introduced one week at a time. For more information visit:

www.stress.parkinsonsrecovery.com

Parkinsons Recovery Memberships involve a variety of support websites that are essential to recovery. A difference mindfulness exercise is posted each week. For more information on Parkinsons Recovery memberships visit:

www.parkinsonsrecovery.org

Of course, the approach that works for many people is to purchase a single volume of the Parkinsons Recovery

Mindfulness program at a time as you have already done! See the introduction for a listing of all nine Parkinsons Recovery Mindfulness volumes.

Thank you for Your Support

On behalf of the thousands of followers of Parkinsons Recovery, I want to thank you for your purchase of this booklet. One hundred percent (100%) of the profits purchases of my books and programs help subsidize the many free services I offer through Parkinsons Recovery -

www.parkinsonsrecovery.com

For information about other products, services and programs visit -

www.parkinsonsrecovery.me

www.ingramcontent.com/pod-product-compliance
Lightning Source LLC
Chambersburg PA
CBHW070244290526
45789CB00004B/1762